Addicted

Addicted

All Rights Reserved

Copyright © Terry Davis

Reproduction in any manner, in whole or in part,
in English or any other language, or otherwise,
without the written permission of the copyright holder is prohibited

For information address
terryd1900@hotmail.com

First Printing 2024

ISBN: 987-0-6459672-2-7

Foreword

As the parents of Michelle, we believe that we need to give our views and opinions on what has happened to our lovely and beautiful daughter.

Firstly, what is Addiction?

Experts tell us, *Addiction is a* <u>neuropsychological</u> *disorder characterised by a persistent and intense urge to use a* <u>drug</u> *or engage in a behaviour that produces natural reward, despite substantial harm and other negative consequences.* It's possible to be addicted to <u>anything</u>!

Our daughter's addiction has had a profound impact on us. Over a period of many years, we have experienced our own mental health issues and financial heartache, which has affected the whole family.

Up to her teenage years, she was a happy and loving daughter with high ambitions, until she met a potential boyfriend in the late 1990s who we thought he was a negative influence on her. We found out some time later, that he did introduce her to start experimenting with drugs such as smoking marijuana. In 2000, she sustained a back injury at work, which later on, required lower back spinal surgery. This was the kick start to pain killers being her friend. In the years following, she started to Doctor and Chemist shop to fulfil her addiction which grew stronger and stronger.

She came back to live with us after years with her boyfriend. After a while, her intake of pain killing drugs increased dramatically. She sought help from a Psychiatrist and all he did was prescribe highly addictive tablets to help with her anxiety and depression. On occasions, she would take the whole box of tablets at once!

We saw her collapse into a coma more than once from overdosing on prescribed pain killers, which was so horrifying and scary not knowing if she would survive. There was one particular time when she collapsed and began to convulse outside her door. I didn't think she was breathing. I was just about to commence resuscitation, when the paramedics walked in the door and took over. She was transported to hospital and placed in a coma while they pumped her stomach of its contents.

She went to a rehabilitation facility for five months and during that time it appeared to be beneficial for her, but that didn't last very long as she went back to her old ways.

Over the last ten years we have reluctantly helped her financially as she found it too difficult to get and hold a job. We both retired a few years ago and are now pensioners on very little income, yet nearly daily, she contacts us for money which we have very little of. We are both extremely worried on how long our funds will last us until the inevitable.

To this day, she still struggles with addiction but tries to manage her thoughts and actions with meditation and yoga.

We both love our daughter very much, but hate the disease she has!

Addicted

2016

It's happened again. Look at me, passed out on the tiled floor. I took too many pills. Why do I do this? It was a strong dose. I just took a heap all at once. I think there were 150 milligrams. I can't remember how many I had taken.

I just remember it being a lot. I look sideways, there's a lot of blood on the floor. I think my hair feels wet. Is it coming from my head? Crap, I must have hit the ground hard. I think I must be concussed. When I became conscious, all I could hear was my dad yelling, "Michelle, Michelle."

"Far out," my dad said. I stopped breathing for a bit, and I was having some kind of fit on the floor. Fuck me! All because of painkillers. I know what this is. This is an overdose. I feel so weak. I don't even know where I am.

I am in the house, I know that. I can't think. Why can't I think properly? I have no energy, and I can't move.

The medics are here now. They bandaged my head. They try to ask me questions. I tried to talk, but I just can't get the words out. I've got nothing and it's scaring me. Oh my God! Why did I do this to myself.

SHIT! What have I done?

Addicted

Hopefully, by writing this book and telling my story, my experiences, the good the bad and the ugly, it might help the message that I really want to bring home is that no matter what's happening for you, how much pain you felt, what you have enjoyed, what people have said or the fact that you have simply hit rock bottom. Despite all these setbacks I want you to know one thing and one thing only. There is always hope. I never used to think there was, but with all that I have been through and all that has happened, there just has to be.

I firmly believe that everything happens for a reason, and I really believe that I am alive for a reason. Perhaps it's to share with all of you just what I have enjoyed and to tell you that you are not alone and that while with all that you have been through, and you might have lost all faith, all courage, or self-respect. I can tell you one thing for sure. You can get this all back. Before rehab I was a very broken woman. I felt like I had nothing. Nothing to live for, I felt lonely and empty for a long time, but then my life did start to turn around. It was a very slow process, but it finally did. I guess I should fill you in on how it all started. To do this I have to go back

Addicted

Back to the Beginning

I guess the first time I started to use a drug, it was alcohol. I was sixteen, that's when it first started. If I was going out to a club or even a party, I would always have some drinks before I went out. I absolutely loved it. Alcohol was a big part of my life for a good four years. When I would party, I would always go hard. I was a teenager, having the time of my life. Alcohol gave me confidence. That was one of the things I liked about it, because I was quite shy and reserved in nature. I guess you could say I was a different person, and I liked the escape. I also loved the attention I got from boys, it made me feel wanted and sexy.

I did the club thing for about a year, then I met my partner. Let's just call him "Mark." At nineteen through a mutual friend. I finally had a boyfriend, so I left the club scene. He was twenty-three. I thought I had found my knight in shining armour. Little did I know I was wrong. I ended up staying with Mark for fourteen years. Mark turned out to be somebody I certainly never wanted in a man. A drug addict. He was addicted to marijuana. I actually found that out in a few months into the relationship. We were dating for about a year until we moved in together. That's when his marijuana use became mine. I started to smoke with him. Then it just became an everyday thing. He would smoke, so I would smoke. So, the years went by and before long I was addicted. I certainly didn't plan for it to happen. It just became a habit. It was always of a nighttime. He would drink as well, beer mostly. When I started to go out with him, I was actually drinking a lot. Every time he would come over, I would drink. One night he got very upset with me and told me I needed to stop drinking or it would be over between us. He gave me an ultimatum. So, at twenty I made the decision to stop. And I stopped.

So, at twenty, we moved in together. And from there on, I became addicted to pot. Everything was going well, but a few years later in 2006, he decided to stop smoking marijuana altogether. So I had to stop, as he was the only one who could get it. I knew no one, so I had to stop too. I had severe withdrawal symptoms from stopping. I started having really bad anxiety, loss of appetite, insomnia and I started to develop really bad lower stomach pain. So I went to the doctor and explained my symptoms and he said, "OK, here's some Valium, some painkillers," so that's what I started to take.

I was in and out of hospital a few times due to my pain, and none of the doctors could find anything wrong with me. They all pretty much said the same thing, it's severe anxiety. So I got some more pills. I kept going back to see my doctor at the time and he just kept on giving me more medications all the time, so during this time, I developed an addiction to pills. From 2006 to 2013 I was using pills and during this time I did go back to smoking marijuana again.

Addicted

But in 2013, I realised I was in a horrible situation, and I realised I wasn't in love with Mark, so I ended up leaving him. I quit him, pills and pot, all on the same night. I was finally free from my abusive, alcoholic, addict partner. I actually detoxed myself from the pills a few weeks before I left. I became clearer headed and that's when I realised I wasn't happy. So, on that night I went to stay with my parents, where I lived with them for six years. Then I started to get codeine from the chemist when it was allowed. Then, a couple of years later, they stopped it. You could only get it on prescription. Then, after these five years of being sober, I ended up relapsing. So for three years I just kept going to different pharmacies. I also started seeing a psychiatrist. He would always end up prescribing Valium and sleeping pills every month I went to see him, which ended up accelerating my addiction.

I put my parents through hell. They would see me out of it all the time. My mom would get upset, my dad got angry and my brother would also get livid with me and not talk to me for two or three days. Not that I blame him. They all just didn't know how to handle my disease, and I'm sure they felt very helpless. To be honest, I really don't want to think about what I did to them and how they felt. It absolutely devastates me, how could I hurt my family like that? I mean, you can't justify that. The only way I know how is to have a disease. A really awful brain disease.

Addicted

So, in 2016 I went to detox for a week. I knew I had to go. Things were not going great. I won't sugarcoat it, detox was hard. The first few days were rough. But the staff was so great and so supportive and even some of the people you meet are awesome because you can relate to one another as you have the same disease. So, I was there for a week, and I would say about day five, things started to get a little easier. I was feeling a bit happier and didn't seem to feel as sluggish. By day seven, I felt great. So, if you just hang in there for a few days, things will start to go in a better direction. It was hard, but I hung in there, got through it, and I just started to feel more comfortable in my own skin

So, I got out, things were going really well, I started walking, going out by myself again. I was just feeling much happier and positive. Then I would say, a couple of months later, I started to feel my back pain again. See, in 2010 I hurt my back by simply just bending over, which resulted in having a herniated disc in my lower back. See, when I was overusing the painkillers, I hardly ever felt the pain. Now, having no painkillers, I was feeling the same pain again, even six years later.

A few weeks later after detox, I went to a Doctor who prescribed me Endone. From there, that was it. My disease was activated. From 2016 to 2018, I was messed up. I needed help. I resisted it for a while. My dad kept on saying, "You have to go to rehab." I rang Lifeline and told the lady my problem and she said, "Your dad is right, you have to go."

Addicted

I hung up on the call, then I made the decision to go to rehab. My dad was obviously happy, but probably more relieved now that I had actually admitted I needed help. It was about three weeks to a month later that I went to rehab.

I do want to talk about my experience of going into rehab, but first I would like to just talk about exactly what addiction is. I think it's very important for people to have knowledge of addiction, as some people are not quite sure of just what it means to be an addict. Some people believe you can help it, and you can stop anytime. Some people don't think addiction is a disease. But as you will see, addiction is definitely a disease. A brain disease

> There are all kinds of addicts.
> We all have pain.
> And we all look for ways
> To make the pain go away

Chapter 1
What is addiction?

Addiction is a brain disease. It is summed up as this;

It is based on two things, genetics and environment, which result in abnormal biology, reflecting in signs and symptoms that follow a different pattern and have a predictable response to treatment. That is a disease.

This disease affects 60% of the population based on genetics. Believe it or not, you can still have the gene and not have an addiction. This has happened.

This disease distorts your motivation, mental health, your need for survival, your clarity, etc. The list goes on. All needs are thrown out of the window. You don't care whether you actually survive, or if you have hurt your family/friends. Your rationality is no longer in existence. All that matters is getting that particular drug or drink. Consequences never enter your mind. You have no fear and are completely selfish. All you want to do is drink or use.

People don't understand how physiology goes wrong. That's why it is a brain disease

Addiction is a disease that affects you physically, mentally, spiritually and emotionally.

Addiction means the individual has no control over the drug they use. They are using it compulsively and there are no consequences to using the drug, but they continue to use it anyway. They are not in control of their actions.

A number of factors contribute to this disease. They can include genetics, environmental stress and personality traits.

People who suffer from addiction may have distorted thinking and behaviours. Changes in the brain's structure and function are what cause people to have cravings, a changing personality, abnormal movements and other behaviours. Brain scan studies have shown changes in the areas of the brain that relate to judgement, decision making, learning, memory and behavioural control.

Individuals that suffer from mental health issues such as depression, bipolar disorder and ADHD are more likely to abuse substances. The reason for this is that a large majority of people try to self-medicate with drugs or alcohol in an attempt to numb the painful symptoms or their disorder.

Drug addiction isn't just about heroin, cocaine or other illegal drugs. You can also become addicted to alcohol, nicotine, opioid painkillers and other legal substances.

At first, you might choose to take a drug because of the way it makes you feel. You may think you can control how much and how often you use it, but over time, drugs change how your brain works. These physical changes can last a long time. They make you lose self-control.

Addicted

Addictive behaviour is the result of a need to self soothe. Anything can become an addiction if done habitually and for the need to feel completely numb. We turn to addiction to escape pain, but the escape perpetuates our pain and begins a dangerous spiral. In reality, we want to kill the pain, and we often engage in other self-destructive behaviour. We forget that psychological pain has a purpose. It is an additive function warning us that something is wrong.

Addiction is when you can't stop. Not when it puts your health in danger. Not when it causes financial emotional and other problems for you or your loved ones. The urge to get and use the drugs can fill up every minute of the day, even if you want to stop.

People who have addictions have distorted thinking, behaviour and body functions. There are changes that happen in the brain's wiring and that is what causes people to have intense cravings for the drug or alcohol, making it hard to stop using.

These substances can cause harmful changes in how the brain functions. These changes can last long after the immediate effects of the drug/intoxication. Intoxication is the intense pleasure, calm, increased senses or a high caused by the drug. Intoxication effects differ between each substance.

Over time, people with addiction build up a tolerance, needing larger amounts to feel the effects.

Illness also, e.g. depression, bipolar anxiety, etc. Mental illness might be present before the addiction or the addiction itself may trigger or make a mental disorder worse.

Addiction can happen to anyone and at any stage of life.

It is important to remember that you are not a bad person. Addiction is a disease.

Addiction is a family disease.

When you are part of a family, decisions that a person makes can influence the other family members. When one family member struggles with addiction, this can negatively affect all the family members by putting them in a state of high stress and anxiety. There are feelings of guilt, shame, anger, confusion, sadness, helplessness and more trouble leading the entire family to increased conflict, isolation and dysfunction.

Everyone suffers

From the closest relative to the most distant, everyone suffers on some level of distress when addiction grips the family. Possible effects of family addition include:

Mental health problems worsen by ongoing stress such as:
- Anger and resentment;
- Anxiety;

- Hopelessness and depression;
- Risky sexual behaviour and promiscuity;
- Shame:
- Isolation;
- Physical health issues resulting from an intense focus on the person using substances rather than focusing on your own needs;
- Financial issues stemming from supporting a loved one's habit, having been stolen from, paying legal fees, and having financial resources needed for housing, utilities and nutrition being spent on drugs and or/ alcohol.

Substance abuse places children in the family at increased risk of ill effects and suffering, like:

- Depression;
- Anxiety;
- Low self-esteem;
- Impaired relationships in the future;
- Higher rates of divorce;
- Increased likelihood of abusing substances themselves;
- Violence; and
- Diminished capacity for learning.

Addicted

Two of the more serious maladaptive interactive patterns to develop in family or addiction are co-dependency and enabling.

Co-dependency is being overly concerned with a family member, while spending little time and energy on your own needs. Co-dependent family members may:

- Have low self-esteem;
- Appear to be very controlling because they do not trust their family member;
- Seem overly flexible to avoid anger and rejection;
- Have oversensitive reactions to problems; and
- Stay loyal and dependent on the person always.

Enabling - the state of constantly working to protect the family member from the natural consequences of substance abuse. By making excuses, bailing their loved ones out of jail, paying for legal fees and otherwise staving off negative consequences, an enabler prevents the family member from experiencing the true cost of their addiction.

Children are not immune to changing the family dynamics. In many situations, roles reverse, and the child begins to take on the caregiving role for their substance-abusing parent. This can create extreme stress for the child, blur the appropriate boundaries and set the child up for difficulty setting healthy boundaries in future relationships. The environment that the child grows up in may also be a factor.

Symptoms of Addiction

- The substance or activity is used in larger amounts or for longer periods of time;
- There is a desire to cut down on use or unsuccessful attempts to do so;
- There is a craving or a strong desire to use the substance or activity;
- Use of the substance or activity disrupts obligations at work, school or home;
- Use of the substance or activity continues, despite the social or interpersonal problems;
- Participation in important social work or recreational activities drops or stops;
- Use occurs in situations where it is physically risky;
- Use continues despite knowing it is causing or exacerbating physical or psychological problems;
- Tolerance occurs, indicated either by the need for markedly increased amounts of the substance; and
- Withdrawal occurs.

The severity of the condition is gauged by the number of symptoms present. The presence of one to three indicates a mild condition; four to five symptoms indicate a moderate disorder. When six or more symptoms are present, this is considered severe.

Effect on Your Brain

Your brain is wired to make you want to repeat experiences that make you feel good. So you are then motivated to do them again and again.

The drugs that may be addictive target your brain's reward system. They flood your brain with a chemical called dopamine. This trick is a feeling of intense pleasure. So you keep taking the drug to chase that high.

When someone develops an addiction, the brain craves the reward of the substance. This is due to the intense stimulation of the brain's reward system. Because of this, many continue to use the substance, therefore creating a host of euphoric feelings and strange behavioural traits. Long term addiction can have severe outcomes, like brain damage, and can even result in death.

The brain regulates temperature, emotions, decision-making, breathing and coordination. This major organ in the body also impacts physical sensations in the body, emotions, cravings and habits.

Drug use interacts with the limbic system in the brain to release strong feel-good emotions, affecting the individual's mind and body. Our brains reward us when we do something that brings us pleasure. Eventually, people take the drug just to feel normal.

As a consequence of drug addiction, the brain rewards itself, meaning it encourages drug addiction, keeping the person in a cycle of highs and lows, on an emotional rollercoaster of feeling desperation and depression when the individual stops. Once someone suddenly does stop, there are harsh mental, physical and emotional results. Withdrawal symptoms are usually stronger for some substances than others.

Drugs are chemicals. When someone puts these chemicals into the body, they tap into the brain's communication system and affect the way the nerve cells send, receive and process information. Different drugs, because of their chemical structures, work differently. We know there are at least two ways drugs work in the brain:

- Interfering in the brain's natural chemical messengers, and
- Over-stimulating the "reward circuit" of the brain.

2017

My back's hurting again today. Oh, how my addiction is so happy about this. In my head, I reasoned with it. I'll say, "I am in pain," which I am. "But stuff it" I say. I'm going to the doctor to get Tramadol. Got it. Went home. I took it. Think the strength I got was 150 milligrams. It's a slow release. I got twenty. Geez, really? Can feel it start to kick in. Bloody strong! Oh no, I've taken too many. So I go into my room. That's all I can remember. I am lying on the floor. Apparently, I had some sort of a fit. I can hear my mother calling out for my father. Don't know what's happening. I'm finding it a bit hard to breathe. The ambulance is here again. Back to hospital again. Another overdose again. All of this as a result of wanting to feel high?

Seriously, what's wrong with me? I need help!

Chapter 2
Why Keep On Taking Drugs/Alcohol?

People continue to drink or take drugs for a lot of reasons - to relax, have fun, socialise, to cope with problems, escape life or to numb a physical/ emotional pain. But see, the thing is, that while you use substances to cope with problems, it doesn't make them go away, it can actually make it worse and may add new problems to the mix. Becoming independent on drugs to cope, instead of getting help or finding positive solutions, can create longer term problems. They think drugs are the solution, but over time, the drugs become the problem. People take drugs because they want something to change in their life.

Some of the reasons people take drugs:
- To fit in;
- To escape or to relax;
- To relieve boredom; and
- To experiment.

Drugs are poisons. The amount taken determines the effect.

A small amount can act as a stimulant (speed you up). A larger amount acts as a sedative (slows you down). An even larger amount poisons you and can kill.

This is true of any drug. Only the amount needed to achieve the effect differs.

Addicted

But many drugs have another consequence: they directly affect the mind. They can distort the user's perception of what is happening around them. As a result, the individual's actions might be odd, irrational, inappropriate and destructive.

This is a very common reason why people keep on taking drugs, and I can relate to this myself. If drugs are so bad and they make you feel awful, the natural thing would be to stop doing it, right? Nearly all addictive people believe that they can stop using drugs/alcohol on their own, and most do try to stop it without seeking treatment. Although some are successful, many attempts result in failure to achieve long term abstinence. Research has shown that long term drug/alcohol abuse results in changes to the brain that continue long after a person stops using drugs or drinking. These drug-induced changes in the way your brain functions can have a lot of behavioural consequences, including the inability to exert control over the impulse to use drugs/drink, regardless of the consequences - the defining characteristics of an addiction.

Understanding that addiction has such a fundamental biological component, might help explain the difficulty of achieving and maintaining abstinence without treatments. Psychological stress from work, family problems, psychiatric illness, pain due to medical problems, social cues (such as encountering individuals from one's drug-using past) or environmental cues (such as encountering streets, objects, or even smells associated with drug abuse) can trigger intense cravings, even without the person's knowledge of them being aware of it.

Any one of these factors can set back sustained absence and make relapse more likely. Research indicates that active participation in treatment is essential for good outcomes and can be beneficial, even in worse addicted individuals.

Drug treatment is intended to help addicts stop compulsive drug seeking and use. Treatment methods can occur in different sorts of settings, take many different lengths of time. Because drug addiction/alcohol is usually a chronic disorder characterised by occasional relapses, short-term, one-time treatment is usually not sufficient. For the majority, treatment is a long-term process that can require multiple interventions and regular monitoring.

Treatments for prescription medication abuse are usually similar to those who are addicted to illicit drugs that affect the same brain systems. For example, buprenorphine, used to treat heroin addiction, can also be used to treat addiction to opioid pain medications. Addiction to prescription stimulants, which affect the same brains systems as illicit stimulants like cocaine, can be treated with behavioural therapies, as there are not yet medications for treating addiction with these types of substances.

Dependence

Most of us will admit that we are dependent on your cars, computers, money, partners or our friends.

One definition of dependence is: a state of relying or on being sustained by something.

When it comes to drug dependence, society can tend to view it as something quite different from these everyday behaviours.

Drug dependence occurs when you need one or more drugs to function. The American Psychiatric Association used to distinguish between dependence and abuse. Abuse was considered the mild or early phase of inappropriate drug use that led to dependence. People view dependence as a more severe problem than abuse.

In my experience, being dependent on drugs will only keep you using. Unless of course, you seek treatment like detox, which will help your body to recover getting off the substance/s. Rehab will help unlock a lot of blocks and different sorts of actions, which in turn are needed to be taken for you to regain your inner strength and mentality.

There is great value in telling your story to others and making sense of the negative events that have shaped us, all the small traumas that led us to feel like we have to escape and turn to addiction in order for us to cope. We can better identify when and why we got triggered and alter our response to these triggers. When we understand the source of our intensified emotions, we feel owned by them. We can then start to feel more secure in ourselves and have stronger relationships with others. In doing so, we reject our desire for escape. Continued use of drugs or alcohol interferes with the motivation and reward chemistry and circuitry, resulting in drug cravings and dependence.

When drug abuse escalates to dependence, treatment can become complicated.

The following are known triggers for substance use disorders:

- Having a family history of addiction;
- Living within an environment where illegal drugs are often used and easy to access;
- Having a history of anxiety;
- Having a history of depression; and
- Having a history of other mental health conditions.

You can often tell if an addiction has turned into dependence by observing the person's behaviour. When a person who is addicted to drugs and hasn't had them for a period of time, this can cause a physical reaction. Physical symptoms of withdrawal occur when the body becomes stressed without the drug. These symptoms include:

- Anxiety;
- Depression;
- Muscle weakness;

- Nightmares;
- Body aches;
- Sweating;
- Nausea; and
- Vomiting.

If left untreated, dependence on drugs can be dangerous. You might increase your drug use as your body adapts to the drugs. This can result in overdose or even death.

Treatment can reverse dependence, but you must want to be treated.

Numbing the Pain

When a person hasn't learned how to use healthy techniques to navigate difficult emotions, they tend to fall into unhealthy emotional patterns of trying to escape our pain and numb ourselves from it. They then use drugs and other behaviours to self-medicate from the emotions they are having a hard time facing. As addicts, we would rather go round the feeling, instead of going through the feeling. It is because we are in patterns of denial, avoidance, secrecy and emotional suppression, all of which cause our pain over time to grow stronger.

When we don't have that healthy technique to navigate our difficult emotions, we tend to fall in unhealthy emotional pain and numb ourselves from it.

Addicted

We turn to our drug of choice, our addictive substances and behaviours, to self-medicate from the emotions we are having a hard time facing. Often, we get caught up in patterns of denial, avoidance, secrecy and emotional suppression, all of which cause our pain to grow stronger over time. What happens to us as we continue to numb or pain?

Many of us have grown accustomed to numbing our pain because as addicts, that is the only way we know how to take away the pain, to not feel and to avoid any feeling that causes us discomfort and pain.

While this solution may seem like a good idea at the time, it actually makes the problems worse, rather than better.

Whatever your drug of choice is, it will alleviate the pain, but the effect will only last as long as you were under the influence. As soon as the alcohol or drug wears off, the emotional pain will come back, probably worse than it was before.

Although escaping the pain by taking drugs may seem like the answer, the only way of truly escaping is by eventually facing your emotional pain and working through it.

There are many strategies that you can use if you want to work through this on your own, including:

- Join a mindfulness, yoga or meditation class. You can find these at your local community centre or through yoga and meditation groups;

- Read self-help books. If you can't afford it, you can try your local library. Books on mindfulness work for any kind of emotional pain; and
- You can see a counsellor who can help you uncover and deal with the emotions that are underlying your addiction.

Getting the Right Medication

Sometimes, emotional and physical pain is caused by a condition such as depression or anxiety disorder. A number of physical conditions can cause emotional symptoms, such as low mood, fatigue and irritability can mirror those of depression.

These are not "normal" emotional reactions and can be effectively treated with the right medications. Anti-depressants are not usually addictive, while anti-anxiety medications can be, and all should only be taken as prescribed.

Anti-depressants should never be stopped abruptly, because of the risk of withdrawal symptoms and possible relapse.

Talk to your doctor if you don't feel like you can manage your emotions on your own, and they will advise you about what type of medication is right for you.

Feels like I am sinking. Going under. My head is in my hands. I feel so alone. Right now, it feels like I am

Addicted

the only person in the world who is drowning. No one can hear me. No one. Should I just scream? What's the point? Don't know which way to turn. This is one of my lowest days. I wish I had some pills to take away the loneliness. Would be nice. They are like my comforter, my best friend. Seriously, how messed up am I? Crying inside. Why won't this go away? God, I need you. Please help me. Take away my pain. I just want my life back. I just wish I had it all together. I want love and to be in love. I just want to be happy inside. Guess it will happen one day. In the meantime, I hope to get back to me. My true self. I want to live. I don't want to die. I want to make it. I choose life. Although yes, the struggle is real, I have to believe that eventually the struggle will be over. I have to keep fighting. Fighting for me. I am alive and I have to believe it's for a reason.

Never give up. That is my motto.

Chapter 3

Emotions

A big part of active addiction is avoiding your emotions. Whether it's drinking or getting high when you feel angry, sad, happy, anxious, frustrated, excited... and so on. Actually, no matter the emotion, all you really want to do is to just feel numb.

While in recovery from addiction, everyone who was once in active addiction finds that ultimately in the end, they have to confront their emotions. You will have to face things that make you feel uncomfortable. I know when I was in rehab, I had to unfortunately feel things that made me feel very uncomfortable. It was like I couldn't hide anymore. I knew that I had to start dealing with these emotions, otherwise there was no other way I could get better than start the healing process. These lists of emotions I'm about to list are all of what I had to start dealing with.

Guilt

In most cases of addiction, it's likely that a lot has gone wrong. Whether your guilt stems from a specific incident or a continued pattern of behaviour, feeling guilty is a natural emotion that plays into your recovery, especially early on, and this feeling can be quite overwhelming. Remember, there is nothing wrong with guilt. But actually feeling some sort of remorse for the actions that may have caused you pain, or to others, can be a form of motivation for change.

What you can do:

You can acknowledge your wrongdoings and try to work on making amends. While some friends or family members may not choose to forgive you, know that that is their choice, not yours, and you can't control other people's reactions. If you feel as though your feelings of guilt are overwhelming, try to talk with a counsellor or a sponsor on how to work towards ways to make amends and to move away from the guilt.

Shame

Shame and guilt can be confused with one another. Shame, however, occurs when you believe that something inherently is wrong with you.

Shame usually leaves us with low self-worth, low self-esteem and the feeling of helplessness. You might feel like you are worthless and are unable to accomplish anything or move forward with your life.

Shame will prevent you from forming relationships, from seeking help, it will trap you in an overwhelming belief that you're meant to feel this way.

What you can do:

Working through and overcoming shame usually does require the help of a counsellor, sponsor or a friend who is in recovery, as well as the support of your loved ones. You can also keep a diary, jotting down all your successes, progress, and your thoughts can be quite therapeutic. Writing down your journey/thoughts can be a great outlet as opposed to letting it build up inside. Ultimately rebuilding your self-esteem is key to battling shame and taking on the goals of recovery.

Worry

Worry is a big one. You can often spend time going over in your head about what I should have done differently, or if only I did it differently instead of doing what I did.

When you spend your time worrying, it's just absolutely pointless. You put a lot of energy into things that you have no control over. You might imagine scenarios that didn't happen or visualise events that will never happen and focus on possible disasters that aren't even really possible.

The truth is we only know what we know at any given moment at the time, and at the time, you reacted the only way you knew how to at that moment, with the knowledge you had at that time, so when you think about it, there really wasn't any other way that you could have reacted.

Life has unfolded a certain way for you so far, and the future will unfold also, regardless of how much you worry about it.

What you can do:

The best way you can overcome worry is by simply focusing on one day at a time, or maybe in some cases, one hour or one task at a time. Sticking close to others who are in recovery, as well as mentors, sponsors and supportive friends and family can help you remain focused on the present, instead of the past or future. When you are able to take hold of that energy, you'll be able to put it towards changing the things that you can.

Resentment

Holding onto resentment is like drinking poison and hoping that the other person gets ill. Hanging onto anger and bitterness towards another person is way more harmful to you than it is to them while you are spending your time dwelling on the hurt, injustice or the pain that another person has caused you to feel. They are more than likely just going about their usual everyday lives, well not even giving you any thought.

What you can do:

Sometimes in life, people do us wrong. They really hurt us. Holding on to your anger or hurt is not going to do you any good. It can only make you feel sick and in fact, it can trigger you to return to your drink or drug of choice. Working towards forgiveness doesn't mean that you're excusing the other person's behaviour, it will allow you to mentally move forward. In order to forgive, you don't need to speak to the other person, especially if you aren't on speaking terms. By making a conscious decision to let go, you will regain time, energy, comfort and most importantly your freedom. Remember you are choosing to let it go for you, not for the other person.

Loneliness

The cycle of loneliness can be overwhelming when you are in active addiction. Those who are new to recovery may have realised that in order to get better, they need to cut ties with old friends who are still using, family members who triggered them, and then completely change their lifestyle. This can be hard and so this can cause deep feelings of loneliness.

Loneliness can make you more vulnerable to triggers and urges, and can keep your mind focused on the negativities in your life. When in active addiction, your best friend may have been addicted to pills or alcohol or other drugs. What is happening is you are actually grieving a loss. It's like somebody close to you has died.

What you can do:

We grow our best when we are connected with others. When I was in rehab, I found that the support I had from other people who became my friends really did help me to heal. I realised that you need people. You need the support. So, as you begin your recovery, it's important to make connections. They are in recovery, too.

Also going to a twelve-step group meeting and being a service to others by volunteering at a local soup kitchen can help you as well.

Look, it just takes time to erase feelings of loneliness. You have to give yourself some time to truly heal. It's just a time thing. Being active and surrounding yourself with support will help you on the road to recovery.

Addiction is a feelings disease. When the emotions you feel become too much, turning to alcohol or drugs can blot them out. Sometimes it's a memory of trauma or abuse that the individual cannot bear, and they have to find something in order to block it out.

When you begin treatment, you reconnect with a whole host of feelings and emotions. If you can think back to being a child and remember your earliest experiences of feeling sad or happy or scared, these feelings seem to take over your entire being until you learn to manage it, and this is much like being in early treatment.

Anxiety and depression are very common among addicts. All we want to do is just literally take a vacation from feeling so bad. It's important to remember that we use because we feel bad, not because we are bad people. It's because you are uncomfortable with what you are feeling.

Addicted

You started to use and abuse drugs or alcohol because of problems affecting firstly, your emotional nature and later, your spiritual nature. These problems have many of their origins in your childhood and adolescence, and they are having an impact on you, here and now. At some point in your past, you begin to achieve relief from these emotional and spiritual problems through a physical solution. You began to use substances or perhaps indulge in an activity that had a pleasurable physical effect on you through your body.

So, it was the physical effect of these substances alcohol or other drugs that make them addictive. Your use became abuse. So you became addicted. The solution you found to your emotional and spiritual problems became a shortcut to emotional peace if not spiritual peace. Therefore you began using the shortcut repeatedly, despite ever-reducing success. Eventually you lost sight of the fact that there is a longer but more effective pathway to emotional and spiritual peace.

As you became physically addicted, you continue to use, despite the harmful physical effects on you. Through your physical senses or intellect, you became aware of that physical harm but continued your addictive behaviour, anyway. That is what addiction is! Your need for the physical pleasure had a greater and more immediate effect on you than your knowledge and awareness of the physical harm.

Your need was sometimes physical when your body protested the lack of the substance on which you have become dependent. At other times, your need was emotional or spiritual when physical withdrawal was no longer a problem that you returned to using anyway. Relapse always followed abstinence.

"We had regained good physical health many times, only to lose it by using again. Our track record shows that it is impossible for us to use successfully."

What started as a physical solution to your problems resulted in a downhill disease affecting you mentally emotionally, physically and spiritually.

"Mentally, we became obsessed with the thought of using, regardless of the consequences. Spiritually, we became totally self-centred in the course of our addiction."

According to the National Institute on Drug Abuse, people begin taking drugs for a number of reasons, including:

- To feel good, feelings of pleasure, "high" or "intoxication;"
- To feel better, relieve stress, forget problems, or feel none;
- to do better, improve performance or thinking; and
- Curiosity and peer pressure or experimenting.

People who are fighting addiction may feel like they have failed to live up to expectations, either their own or those of loved ones, and that their life is a disappointment. They might also be sad about opportunities they have missed out on, because of their addiction. Whatever the reasons, their lives can be filled with sadness.

No matter how simple or complex the perceived threats are, they are all very real to the person feeling them. Fear can negatively impact the thinking and decision making of people with addiction and loved ones alike and can lead to irrational and impulsive behaviour.

Chapter 4

The Withdrawal Stage

Withdrawal is also known as detox. It's when you cut out or cut back on using alcohol or other drugs. You may have developed a physical or psychological dependence on a drug or both. Symptoms experienced during withdrawal can be mild or severe depending on:

- How long you've been using;
- What drugs;
- Age;
- Physical health;
- Psychological characteristics; and
- Method of withdrawal.

Physical Dependence

This is when you have been taken off a drug for a while and your body has come to rely on it to feel normal. Your body is now used to functioning with the drug in your system, so if the drug isn't taken then, withdrawal symptoms start to appear.

Psychological Dependence

This is when you believe you need the drug in order to function. You believe that you need it for specific situations, like being social at a party, or to unwind after work, or it could be all the time.

What Can I Expect?

While your body is getting used to functioning without the drug, you can experience a range of symptoms from minor to serious. Withdrawal feels like the opposite of the drug. For example, when you are withdrawing from a depressant like alcohol, you might feel restless and agitated, or experience tremors. These symptoms vary between people and between drugs.

Cravings

Cravings for the drug happen because your brain has learned that the easiest and quickest way to feel better is by using the drug. It's because this was your way of dealing with problems and avoiding bad feelings. It's a learnt behaviour.

The cravings come and go. Sometimes they may be weak and sometimes very strong. But remember, cravings do not last. Managing cravings is very important in the long term, because as mentioned, they do come and go and you might even still feel them occasionally, even years after you have stopped using. Learning to manage cravings involves distraction and relaxation techniques such as reading, watching a movie, meditating or exercising. I actually find that exercising is the best one you can do, as it releases chemicals in the brain that make you feel happy. It also helps to get rid of chemicals that make you feel stressed and anxious. It also improves your quality of sleep.

It might help to remind yourself that your brain has learned this pattern of thought overtime, and you can retrain it to follow a new pattern.

Medication can sometimes be used to help treat withdrawal symptoms from certain drugs.

Time

Withdrawal can last from a few days to a few weeks, but some symptoms like cravings can take longer. How long depends on factors like:
- The type of drug;
- How long you have been using it;
- Your general health; and
- The setting you choose to withdraw in.

Is Withdrawal Safe?

You may need medical supervision to have a safe withdrawal. When I had to go through withdrawal, I found that a detox centre I went to was the best and safest way to go about it. You received 24/7 care, and you always have that support when you need it. It's important to discuss withdrawal with your doctor.

Where Can I Go?

You need a safe and supportive environment when withdrawing. Have a discussion with your doctor, or a drug and alcohol service for advice on which setting will be the best for you.

Home Based Withdrawal

Usually it is provided with a team including your doctor or a support person like a family member or a good friend. If your withdrawal won't be complicated, this might be a good choice.

Outpatient Withdrawal

If you don't need to be admitted to a residential service, then this is a good choice. It involves one-on-one consultations with a health professional over a short period of time, and you also receive ongoing counselling and support.

Residential Withdrawal

This usually involves a five to ten day stay in a residential withdrawal unit or hospital with staff available 24 hours a day. They will help you during your withdrawal and also to avoid relapse. Some units won't allow you to have any contact with your family, call the partners or friends for a while. This is to help you focus on your treatment instead of worrying about what is happening at home. It also helps you to keep out of contact with other people who are using drugs as this can cause cravings.

What To Expect From Drug Withdrawal

Withdrawal from alcohol or drugs comes with various unpleasant symptoms. These symptoms vary in severity and depend on several factors. Which drug you were addicted to plays the largest role, but personal factors like genetics and metabolism make a difference, too.

Symptoms of withdrawal can begin within a few hours of your last use of the drug, or there might take even days to appear. They could last anywhere from days to weeks. In cases of severe addiction to certain drugs, long term symptoms could be experienced for months.

It is easy to relapse while you are getting sober. This is because of the uncomfortable and even painful symptoms of withdrawal. This is why I strongly advise it is best to go to a medical detox centre, where they can monitor you closely and ease discomfort and treat potentially dangerous withdrawal symptoms.

After you detox, a treatment programme, like partial hospitalisation, or intensive outpatient, treats long term withdrawal symptoms while teaching you how to live a sober life.

Withdrawal symptoms usually have several stages. They include:

- An acute withdrawal period, when the symptoms are the most intense. This lasts anywhere from a couple of days to a week;
- A prolonged withdrawal period after physical symptoms subside. This includes long term symptoms like depression and cravings; and

- A protracted withdrawal period, when symptoms are at their worst, then start to fade.

Common Withdrawal Symptoms

The concept of tolerance helps us understand why withdrawal symptoms happen. It doesn't tell us why you might experience certain symptoms and someone else withdrawing from the same drug may not. A couple of things determine which effects you will experience like:

- the type of drug used; and
- How high your tolerance is.

Some similarities exist among withdrawal symptoms from all substances:
- **Rebound effects**: these are symptoms that the drug was originally designed to control. They arise in full force once you stop taking the drug. For example, you may feel pain during an opioid withdrawal, anxiety during benzodiazepine withdrawal, or lethargy during a stimulant withdrawal;
- **Decreased tolerance**; this occurs rapidly during drug withdrawal. It can be dangerous if you relapse because you might overdose due to your reduced tolerance.
- **Depression;** a lack of motivation or inability to experience pleasure are quite common effects

of withdrawal. *"Anhedonia"* is the inability to feel happiness. It happens with other people in recovery whose brains have been hijacked to produce too much dopamine, the feel-good chemical. In the absence of so much dopamine, people often feel like they can't be happy.

- **Changes to the automatic nervous system**; these symptoms include:
  1. Irregular heartbeat;
  2. Irregular breathing; and
  3. Changes in blood pressure.

More symptoms of withdrawal include:

- changes in appetite;
- changes in mood;
- congestion;
- fatigue;
- irritability;
- muscle pain;
- nausea;
- runny nose;
- sleeping difficulties;
- sweating;
- tremors; and
- vomiting.

More severe symptoms such as hallucinations, seizures and delirium might also occur in some circumstances. The type of drug, the amount you were taking, the amount of time you were taking it and the dosage, all have an effect on the type and severity of the symptoms you may experience.

2019

So, I have now moved out of home. I'm now renting a room and my own private bathroom in a three-bedroom townhouse with a single father who is a couple of years older than me. His son only stays every second weekend. Thank God I get to keep my cat, Max. He has another cat here, so luckily, he likes cats.

What should be a fresh start, hasn't quite turned out that way. I'm still using. Taking pills. All sorts, sleeping pills, painkillers, Valium and so on. I feel horrible. I was so out of it one night thank God my roommate wasn't at home, that I walked really hard into the fence and really hurt my nose. I've still been using all year. I mean, I went to rehab last year to get clean and get help. That did work while I was up there, but then you came out and you're back at your home again. Back to reality. I feel ashamed, depressed and very lost. I know it's not 100% my fault because I have a disease, but the same time you really think you're a piece of crap. Like a failure. I just really don't know what to do at this point. All I want to do is numb my depression. But most of all done by loneliness. I just feel alone.

www.ingramcontent.com/pod-product-compliance
Lightning Source LLC
Chambersburg PA
CBHW071845290426
44109CB00017B/1933